S0-DRR-881

LIFTING THE VEIL OF SILENCE

LIFTING THE VEIL OF SILENCE:
SPIRITUAL HELP FOR HEARING LOSS

Lifting the Veil of Silence is an excellent book that fills a niche that has been largely vacant in the literature on hearing loss. All of us who have hearing loss and those who relate to us on a regular basis are aware of the stress produced by the communication difficulties. These difficulties and the negative emotional reactions to them often occur on a daily basis and result in fatigue, a tendency to retreat, and negative self-valuations. All too often we see people who feel helpless and hopeless regarding their ability to continue to function in the social world. Too often, these negative self-valuations that lead to social isolation and despair result from pessimistic thoughts that may not correspond to the reality of the individual's situation. Gloomy, pessimistic thoughts about one's situation are not likely to lead to efforts to improve that situation, resulting in a self-fulfilling cycle of defeat "negative thoughts and feelings" and further defeat.

One effective way of breaking this cycle is to change the way one perceives his or her situation by looking for the positive aspects of one's situation and focusing all of their attention on those qualities while being realistic about the negatives. Affirmations are very helpful tools in achieving a realistic, yet positive appraisal of one's life situation. I've seen them work for others and myself with life-changing results.

This book takes a spiritual perspective on affirmations and offers helpful guidelines for adopting and applying them in one's daily life. I think it is a welcome addition to the information currently available on learning to live with hearing loss and that many people will not only benefit from reading this book, but will enjoy it as well.

SAMUEL TRYCHIN, PH.D.
Psychologist, Educator,
Author of the *Living with
Hearing Loss* series

Susan Roberts treats us to a highly compassionate, spiritual experience of her mother's hearing loss. It is as much about an exquisite, heart-felt portrait of a mother-daughter relationship, as it is about the ripple effects of hearing loss on other family members. A well-written, poignant gift.

MICHAEL A. HARVEY, PH.D.
Author of *Odyssey of Hearing Loss:
Tales of Triumph* and
*Listen with the Heart:
Relationships and Hearing Loss*

Susan Roberts has given us an insightful look at hearing loss in terms simple enough to apply to our everyday experience. With so many Americans living longer, we will doubtless encounter more hearing-impaired people than any generation in history. We all need to know more about hearing loss and what we can do. Medical science can help, but healing often comes as much from an improved attitude as better technologies. The religious teachers of humanity have always told us a positive outlook can conquer any perceived limitation. *Lifting the Veil of Silence* will help people develop a deeper understanding, compassion, and openness to the possibilities which still abound, even after hearing loss.

REV. THOMAS SHEPHARD,
Unity Magazine

He who has ears to hear, let him hear!

—JESUS

LIFTING THE VEIL OF SILENCE

Spiritual Help for Hearing Loss

SUSAN L. ROBERTS

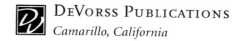
DeVorss Publications
Camarillo, California

Lifting the Veil of Silence
Copyright © 2005 by Susan L. Roberts

All rights reserved. No part of this book may be reproduced,
stored, or transmitted in any form without permission in
writing from the publisher, except by a reviewer who may
quote brief passages for review purposes.

ISBN: 0875168132
Library of Congress Control Number: 2004116135
First Edition, 2005

Affirmations on page 38 are reprinted from
You Can Heal Your Life by Louise Hay, 1984
Hay House Inc, Carlsbad CA

DeVorss & Company, Publisher
P.O. Box 1389
Camarillo CA 93011-1389
www devorss.com

Printed in the United States of America

PUBLISHER'S NOTE

The author is not a physician, nor has she been trained professionally in the medical field of or relating to hearing or the loss of hearing. This book and the author's website (www.susanlroberts.com) is not meant to be a substitute for individualized medical evaluation, advice, care, or recommended treatment from a qualified, licensed health professional. The author or publisher do not recommend any specific treatment, taking supplements, medications or implementing dietary or behavioral programs/changes without first consulting your personal physician and/or therapist.

Although many individuals have expressed their agreement with the material in this book, what the author is proposing is a theory that has yet to be accepted and endorsed by the medical community in general.

The author and publisher disclaim any liability arising directly or indirectly from the use of this book. Statements made by the author about products, processes, treatment methods represent the views and opinions of the author only and in no way do they constitute a recommendation or endorsement of any product or treatment by the publisher.

The author provides in her book, website and other materials several other websites that may be of further interest to readers. The author and publisher make no representation or warranty as to the value, accuracy or completeness of the information these sites contain, and therefore, specifically disclaim any liability for any information contained on, or omission from such referenced websites. References to these websites in this author's materials are not to be viewed in any way as an endorsement of these websites, or of the information they contain, by either the author or the publisher.

I dedicate this book to my Mother, Jean.

Contents

FOREWORD

ifting the Veil is written from my personal point of view. Even though I can hear clearly, I refer to hearing loss inclusively using "we" and "our." I may not know precisely what it's like not to hear, but I do know exactly what it feels like not being heard. Hearing loss is a community loss. When one person is affected, many others are affected as well. Ideally both the person with hearing loss and his or her circle of family and friends change their behaviors to accommodate the loss and remain connected. Spiritually the connection cannot be broken but sometimes our humanness makes it seem so.

Many people impacted by hearing loss do not feel supported in their experience. They are often quick to feel bad, guilty or apologetic for the "inconvenience" they feel they impose on others. Words like *bad, guilt,* and *apology* are terms that describe a human experience but in the realm of Spirit there is no judgment or opposition. For example, when a boulder falls into a river, the water naturally flows around the boulder. The river doesn't "get mad" at the boulder; the boulder doesn't apologize to the river for inconveniencing its flow. The river naturally adapts its flow around the boulder and continues. When we respond to hearing loss from our spiritual self, we create ways to remain connected. Our spiritual experience is one of connection. These words of separation emphasize how much we have lost touch with our spiritual side. I chose to write this book using the inclusive "we" and "our" to emphasize our connection and lessen the appearance of separation.

The Birth of This Book

aised by a mother with severe hearing loss, I have experienced what it's like to live in a world with someone who cannot hear well. About six years ago my mother accidentally discovered a local chapter of SHHH (Self Help for Hard of Hearing People). She found people who were like her and who understood her frustrations. Acknowledging her disability and learning she wasn't the only one with a hearing loss, after nearly fifty years of feeling alone, she became energized. Through SHHH she found a coping skills training class. Transformed by what she learned, she co-coordinated a statewide SHHH conference, a task that, prior to the training she never would have considered doing.

I volunteered at the conference registration table where I spoke with dozens of people with hearing loss. By mid-day I felt an awareness stir within me as I looked over the sea of people. It occurred to me the behaviors I saw were similar to my mother's. They "snapped and barked" when they spoke; they used choppy sentences;

they'd complete a sentence they never introduced. They did all the things my mother did that exasperated me. Deep within my body I felt a shift, a freeing up, an opening. For the first time in my life I started to separate her physical hearing loss from her spiritual self.

Knowing I had more to learn, I read books on hearing loss. I was shocked when I learned my mother could hear only parts of words and parts of sentences. We had never discussed it in our family. Suddenly I understood that all her life she'd been struggling with filling in the missing sounds, which generally meant guessing at what was said—or giving up. Like most people, I thought hearing loss meant the volume had just been turned down. I didn't understand that her choppy sentences resulted from the choppy sentences she received. I didn't understand that the abrupt "barking" was how sounds came across in her world: she does not hear sounds off in the distance; she only becomes aware of them when they are nearby and loud enough to be heard. They are abrupt to her. Like most people I had lived with the assumption that hearing aids "fixed" her hearing. Even though I knew she missed things, I didn't associate it with her hearing loss.

Once I understood the impact of hearing loss on her life, I began separating her from the disability. This allowed me to see her for who she is, and not as the person struggling to hear. I accepted that much of the behavior that had bothered me resulted from her hearing loss. I now could see and accept her Spirit self. While reacting to her outward behavior, I had missed connecting with her on a spiritual level. Rarely noticing her inner goodness, I had missed feeling the abundant love and joy that is her essence. Waves of healing pulsed through my body as I separated my mother's hearing loss experience from her as a person.

A deep sadness overcame me when I accepted that most people with hearing loss will forever miss communications around them. Hearing aids, at best, improve understanding but do not bring back 100% hearing. Lip reading combined with hearing aids can further improve understanding but some words and sounds will always be missed. In even the most accommodating situations, conversations will not be fully heard.

To deal with these disturbing thoughts I sought comfort and insight from my spiritual studies. I found hope in the New Thought spiritual principle that our thoughts and beliefs manifest as our experience: "Thoughts held in mind produce after their kind." Limiting thoughts keep us from the full experience that life can offer us. Could people with hearing loss be helped by this insight?

In the course of my spiritual unfoldment, I trained to be a chaplain. Since many chaplains serve the elderly who are often hard of hearing, I volunteered to share with my classmates tips on how to improve communications with people with hearing loss. In preparing and delivering the training, I had a second spiritual breakthrough.

As a child I always longed for my mother's love yet had learned it would not be there when I needed it. Because of her hearing loss, she did not always respond to my needs to be nurtured, or she responded with choppy, unloving-like words. In my world, she was not there for me. Her inability to hear and all the missed spoken messages reinforced my belief that she did not love me. I learned to close myself off to love, expecting it not to be there. In a flash I understood that blaming my mother for not loving me, I had turned over to her my ability to experience love. Understanding what I had done, I released the energy holding on to that belief and reclaimed my power. For the first time in my adult life I felt powerful. I stood straighter, I squared off my shoulders, and I felt a confidence I had never felt before. I felt loved and loving.

Three weeks after reclaiming my power, I became employed by Agency for Hearing. With love and power flowing within me I began a quest to see my mother's true self without her hearing loss. Five months later, the prayers and affirmations in this book literally wrote themselves: I sat at my computer to write healing prayers for people with hearing loss and four hours later, with ease, the affirmations were completed. I wrote the affirmations seeing my mother as her Spirit self, not as her hearing loss. As I reread the affirmations, I could feel the barriers I had experienced with my mother crumble.

As I write this, I see that the message in this book is the best gift I can give her—that she is whole and complete and she is not her hearing loss. I share these prayers and affirmations with others who experience hearing loss and who may have believed themselves to be less than a perfect Child of God. We are not our hearing loss; we are spiritual beings.

Love and blessings,
Susan

Hearing Facts

Twenty-eight million Americans, or one out of every ten, have hearing loss.

52% of those with hearing loss are working age adults (18–64).

43% of those with hearing loss are seniors (65+).

Currently there are more adults aged 45–64 with hearing loss (10 million) than there are seniors aged 65+ (9 million).

The myths and the silence surrounding hearing loss are changing. People with hearing loss are becoming more mainstream and part of our consciousness. Television shows are featuring main characters with hearing loss (i.e. Sue Thomas in *FBEye* and *CSI*), commercials are featuring hearing loss, (i.e. a Disney commercial features a young girl getting Mickey ears for her grandfather "whose ears aren't what they used to be") and celebrities are openly sharing they have a hearing loss (Ronald Reagan, Bill Clinton, Rush Limbaugh, former Miss America Heather Whitestone McCallum, Halle Berry, and many others). Having a hearing loss and wearing a hearing aid is becoming more acceptable.

Hearing is one of the five senses through which we communicate with our world. The loss of our ability to hear monumentally transforms our life. This book is designed to give us tools to improve our experience of hearing loss. Through working with people with hearing loss, I noticed that those who have the best attitude about their hearing loss also understand it on a spiritual level. Those who draw upon their spiritual understanding seem to open their minds to opportunities that improve their situation. They see beyond their loss and accept it as a new part of their life with new challenges to solve. They accept their loss as an opportunity to learn and continually seek ways in which they can grow from the experience. If you have a hearing loss, the affirmations in this book can help broaden and deepen your spiritual awareness of the loss.

Healing depends on listening
with the inner ear. . . .

—MARION WOODMAN

LIFTING THE VEIL OF SILENCE

CHAPTER **1**

What's Happening to Me?

O n average it takes seven to ten years after we have admitted we have a hearing loss before we do something about it. Seven to ten years can be a long, frustrating time for a spouse, friends and coworkers to deal with our hearing loss. It can be a long and frustrating time for those of us with the loss. Not understanding what we are going through leads to increased miscommunications, continual repeating, and short tempers. The great length of time before we act to improve our situation is a result of three phenomena: we don't realize we are not hearing everything; we associate hearing loss with negative images and don't want to confront our beliefs (i.e., change); and we are going through a natural grieving process.

If we don't know what we're missing, we don't miss it. Because hearing loss happens gradually, we don't realize we are not hearing things. For instance, we don't notice we're not hearing the lawn sprinklers. We don't notice we are not hearing the refrigerator hum. We may not even notice our spouse calling us from another room. We literally don't miss anything and aren't aware we have a loss. Often it is our spouse, friend or coworker who suggests we may have a hearing loss and brings it to our attention. Only when gently confronted do we become aware that we can no longer hear leaves rustle or the dog panting in the summer heat. For example, I have a friend whose spouse had been hinting he may have a hearing loss, but he thought she was crazy and brushed aside her comments. One day, when the two were hiking in the woods a deer jumped up and scuttled off. He had heard nothing—until his partner screamed. He turned to see the deer jump through the brush, and at that moment he knew he could not hear.

Unfortunately we as a society have several negative beliefs regarding hearing loss. We see it as a sign of aging and no longer being productive in society. Our western culture is so youth oriented that we see aging — a natural phase of life—as grim and undignified. When we associate hearing loss with aging, death or some related image, we tend to deny our loss in an effort to resist becoming what we fear. Others of us associate hearing loss with being "broken," no longer "perfect," and feel unworthy. We fear that we will be discarded, just as a broken toy is thrown away. We feel shame for not being as good as we used to be. Rather than confront our beliefs, we deny the hearing loss.

Also, because hearing loss is not visible, we tend to discount its importance; we minimize its impact on our lives and pretend it doesn't exist. Communication experts tell us that 40% of our communication with others is conducted through voice, tone, pace, pitch and rate of speech, all transferred through our auditory system. Another 10% of our communication is expressed through words so up to 50% of our communication comes through our ears. (Body language, seen through our eyes, accounts for the other 50%.) It's easy to understand how devastating blindness would be: not seeing is 50% of our experience with others. But hearing loss is the other 50% and can be equally devastating.

> ". . . after a lifetime in silence and darkness, to be
> deaf is a greater affliction than to be blind. . . .
> Hearing is the soul of knowledge and information
> of a high order. To be cut off from hearing is to
> be isolated indeed."
>
> —HELEN KELLER

To continue the illusion that all is well, we often play a dangerous game of bluffing in which we "pretend" to hear. Our self-esteem is lowered when we hide and lie. Most of the time others know something is not right anyway and an uncomfortable space begins to form. As it becomes obvious we aren't hearing

everything, we are seen as less capable, less reliable
or, to some, downright stupid when errors are made.
It's a dangerous strategy for our self esteem and po-
tentially harmful to relationships.

The third reason the denial phase takes seven to
ten years is that we go through a natural grieving
process for our loss. Many years ago Elisabeth Kübler-
Ross researched the death and dying process and identified specific phases we process through when faced
with a loss. Studies have since shown that these phases
occur for any loss, although especially for major losses
such as death, divorce, loss of a job, a major move, a
child leaving home. When faced with a physical disability where we can no longer do what we once took for
granted, we experience this grieving process. The phases, in no particular order, include denial, bargaining,
anger, depression, and acceptance. We tend to move
among these phases an indeterminate number of
times and for an indeterminate length of time until we
complete the grieving process.

HOW DOES THE GRIEVING PROCESS
AFFECT ME?

We each handle our grief differently. Some just need
time to sort through it; some need to talk it out with a
friend, spouse or even a therapist. Some will move

through it quickly, while others will take several months or even years. Commonly the first phase is denial. When we lose our hearing gradually, it's common for denial to be the first phase and often the longest phase. With many of us it is the spouse, friend or coworker who first notices the hearing loss. Generally it takes many situations before they finally conclude that their spouse, friend, or coworker must not be hearing everything. When they bring the missed communication to our attention, our common response is, "Well, then speak up, you're mumbling!" As we lose our hearing we begin to hear spoken words as "blurred" or muffled.

As the hearing loss becomes worse, we are forced to ask others to repeat themselves. Without noticing, we may ask several times in each conversation for phrases to be repeated. But, more often than not, rather than put out the extra energy, we tend to give up on communicating with others. This spirals quickly into isolation, which only worsens matters. I watched one woman deny she had a hearing problem for years, while at the same time in a women's group where she could not hear, she continually requested that they please speak up. The natural process of denial, however, strains relationships and tends to isolate us from people. Denial is a frustrating phase, both for us and for those around us.

In the denial phase, we may feel "numb" and out of touch with others and on some days barely able to place one foot in front of the other. It's as if we are in shock—and we are. Those of us whose hearing loss showed up suddenly probably moved directly into shock. We could not believe it was happening to us. We attempted to "shake it off," but it stayed. Because the hearing loss was sudden we rushed to a doctor to assess our hearing. When we were told we had a loss, especially a permanent loss, we may have remained in shock. Those of us whose hearing loss occurred gradually also went through a shock phase, but it may have been processed internally and spread out over time while we adjusted psychologically to the change.

Anger is another phase we experience when we lose our hearing. Anger often covers the hurt we feel beneath. Our natural instincts tell us to fight to protect ourselves when we have been wronged (hurt). The anger is motivated by the hurt or pain we're not ready to fully express. Some who like to fight will stay in this phase for a long time. But there is no one to fight. There is no one to blame. Some of us may relate our loss to a former occupation and blame ourselves for choosing that occupation or blame the company for allowing the unsafe conditions. But unless we want to stay in the past forever, we must eventually face the present and let ourselves feel the pain of the loss. Once we do so, we can move on.

At some point we may want to negotiate with God, a physician, or our spouse or friend. In the bargaining phase we feel we can give something up in exchange for having our hearing returned. We bargain to keep what has been ours. But our hearing is gone. Many of us hold in the sadness, not expressing it out loud, hoping the hearing loss is not real and will go away. In time most of us, accepting that we cannot bargain to get our hearing back, allow ourselves to feel the sadness and pain, and move on.

Depression is the phase in which grief, sadness, and pain are felt. Hearing loss is a situation-specific depression, similar to the depression associated with the death of a spouse, the loss of a job, or moving from an old neighborhood. Although not comfortable, depression is common and a natural phase through which we move. Occasionally normal depression turns into a clinical depression and requires professional intervention. Many years ago I read a definition for depression with which I resonated and it has served me well: "Depression occurs when you can't be who you were meant to be." With hearing loss, we can no longer hear or participate in our world as we know it; we can no longer be who we are. When we are limited in our expression with others, it's natural to feel depressed. As we work through pain, shock, anger and other emotions about our loss, we move through this phase. Our Spirit self needs time to process and assimilate the changes. (If we suspect the depression may be more than a situational depression or if it lasts longer than is normal for us, it's best to get professional help. The hearing loss may be a trigger connected with a deeper limiting belief.)

Those of us who have a sudden loss associated with a disease or injury tend to move into the grieving phase with greater ease. Those of us who have permission to feel and express pain will tend to move through it with greater ease. And those of us who were taught not to express our emotions may avoid feeling the pain and remain in the other phases longer before entering the grieving process.

Once we allow ourselves to express the intense emotions associated with our loss, we will move into an acceptance phase. After we have worked through the pain, hurt, anger, and grief, we are ready to deal with the loss and get on with our lives. We take positive action to find ways to best live with the hearing loss: we visit a doctor, read information on hearing loss, check into getting hearing aids, and investigate options to maximize our communications with others in spite of our hearing loss. We speak of our loss with our doctor, spouse, and friends; we may even seek out a support group where we can share with others who have a hearing loss. (See, What Else Can I Do to Support My Hearing Loss on page 85) This is the phase we—as well as our spouse, friends, and coworkers—wait for and celebrate; for action relieves our frustration and feelings of helplessness.

Remember, most of us will move in and out of these phases before moving beyond them. One day we may be in denial, then slip into anger, then acceptance, then back into denial or bargaining and then back into acceptance. We are processing these changes and preparing for the acceptance phase. The process takes time.

In our Western culture many of us are taught that when something is "broken" we replace it or fix it. Frequently with minimal research, we purchase hearing aids to replace or fix our hearing, thinking it will return like before. But we soon find out that we can no longer hear sounds as we once could. Hearing aids are not eyeglasses; they are aids. They "aid" hearing, not repair it. When we cannot fix the loss, we get angry at the doctors, the hearing aid dispensers and sometimes ourselves. In any case, the hearing aids often go into a drawer and remain there while we continue our grieving process. Sometimes hearing aids never make it out of the drawer. As we move through the grieving process and begin to focus on what we have (versus what we don't have), we'll pull these hearing aids out of the drawer and give them another chance.

WHAT'S HAPPENING TO MY EARS?

In layperson's terms, healthy hearing occurs when sound waves entering the outer ear vibrate the ear drum which vibrates the middle ear stirrup/anvil/hammer bones (the smallest bones in our body), sending vibrations through the fluids in the inner ear cochlea. In the cochlea, tiny hairs sway in fluids and through those hairs the signals transfer to the nerves and into the brain. The brain interprets the signals giving meaning to the sounds heard. We actually "hear" in the brain.

There are three kinds of hearing loss. A "conductive" hearing loss is when something breaks down in the middle ear: broken bones, punctured ear drum, excessive earwax, or infection. Many conductive hearing losses can be repaired or at least improved. Most hearing losses, however, are "sensori-neural." When the tiny chochlea hairs break off, they no longer send signals to the brain. No longer receiving certain frequencies, the connections in the brain for those frequencies will disappear. If a hearing aid restores those sounds early in the hearing loss process, it takes only a few weeks to re-activate those connections so the brain can correctly interpret the sounds. If a hearing aid is used after several years of not hearing certain frequencies, the brain will take longer to re-activate the connections. Some believe the connections may never fully return. This is one reason why it's important to get hearing aids sooner, rather than later. The third kind of hearing loss is mixed, meaning it's some combination of both conductive and sensori-neural losses.

When we use hearing aids for the first time, we will go through an adjustment process. The sounds we hear will be different from sounds heard in natural hearing. Immediately everything will probably sound too loud as we've grown accustomed to muffled sounds. Especially with analog hearing aids, all sounds are amplified and sounds we haven't heard for a while will seem terribly loud. I've heard people comment on the loudness of the turning signals in their car or footsteps on uncarpeted floors. Those sounds have always existed before, but we had trained our brain to tune them out and we didn't hear them. We have to allow time for our brain to re-adjust to tuning out background sounds again. Also, especially if years have passed, the brain has lost connections and can no longer "hear" certain sounds. The human brain will go through another change process to re-learn sounds. It needs time to adjust to receiving signals and correctly interpreting the sound. We must be prepared to practice hearing just as we practiced learning to ride a bike, giving ourselves time to adjust and to let our brain re-establish the connections. Many factors enter into how long the brain takes to adjust. Most people will notice improvements within weeks and continue to use the hearing aids until their brain has maximized the connection. An unpleasant aspect of hearing loss for some of us is that sounds heard through a hearing aid sound more mechanical. Some describe them as "tinny" or "metallic." This is also something to which the brain will adjust.

At first we may feel tired after being around others. When we cannot hear all sounds, our brain works double-time to piece together clues to fill in the missing sounds and make sense of the message. We work in a heightened-hearing mode. This can be exhausting. Designed for emergencies, (i.e., when the lights go out in the house and we have to "hear" our way to safety) functioning regularly in this mode tires us quickly. One man who worked as a bank manager related that he felt guilty for taking a private lunch every day and not joining the staff or taking customers to lunch, an expected activity in the small town where he worked. I quickly assured him that eating lunch alone was a wise choice. It's common to feel tired after being around people, especially when we are not used to their communication nuances. We need to plan rest periods when we know we'll be around crowds or with strangers.

I have conveyed some information here relating to hearing loss in order to lay a foundation or framework before discussing the spiritual aspects of hearing loss including how affirmations can help you to improve your hearing. Your public library, bookstore, local support group, or the Internet can all provide you with additional information. If you do not understand your hearing loss, you need to ask your doctor or hearing aid specialist to explain it to you. If you need help dealing with it emotionally, you can seek out a support group or talk with a friend or therapist. A counselor who knew of my work had a client who came in for depression. She quickly identified that he had a hearing loss and she referred him to a community clinic and a coping skills class. He wrote that the class helped him finally to understand what was happening to him. He purchased hearing aids and was no longer depressed. Knowledge is a key factor when adjusting to hearing loss. We need to learn as much as we can about its causes and treatment. Another key factor is how we approach it spiritually. The use of affirmations can have a positive impact on your experience of hearing loss.

CHAPTER 2

Tell Me About Affirmations and How They Can Work for Me

The words we say to ourselves and others about our hearing loss or its impact on us highly influence our experience of hearing loss. Time and again I've seen individuals with the same level of hearing loss have incredibly different experiences. Some associate the loss with aging or death and turn old overnight. Others view the loss as another "strike against them" and express anger toward their loss and/or themselves. Some feel they have a dark cloud over them and are frustrated and bitter. Yet others, with identical or greater hearing losses, see it as just an obstacle to overcome and they resume most of their regular activities with what seem to them minor accommodations. What we say to ourselves and how we express our inner beliefs determine our experience.

WHAT ARE AFFIRMATIONS AND
HOW DO THEY WORK?

Affirmations identify what we want in our life. The words we use call forth or create our future. If we repeat, "I can't hear—I am no good," we will become exactly that, no good. Obeying our words, our mind focuses on "can't hear" and shuts down other forms of communicating as well as hearing; we soon believe we are "no good," often feeling sorry for ourselves. On the other hand, we can use affirmations to our benefit and call forth good into our life: "I am healthy; I communicate well; I am loved." Now our mind focuses on ways to be healthy, ways to communicate, and ways to love and be loved. The words we use prepare our mind for the outcome we expect. The universe—God—gives us what we affirm. We create our outcomes.

Affirmations are written in the present tense. Using the phrases "I am" or "I have" call forth energy to manifest what we affirm. We live and have our power in the present. We have no power in the future; it hasn't happened yet. We have no power in the past; we can't relive the past. We only have power in the moment. We can only do something now.

Affirmations can be effective if spoken out loud, thought "out loud" in the mind or written. Some of us who are not auditory in nature and who can concentrate deeply on the affirmations will have long-lasting results using affirmations in our mind. Others of us give more credibility to spoken words so speaking words out loud may be more effective. Some of us draw upon our natural gift of power when we use our voice and speak the affirmations. Others of us need to see them written and may have better results writing the words. Any of these approaches, or any others, can be effective. The more important aspect of using affirmations is to choose a method that works for us and to repeat our affirmations earnestly and consistently until they take hold of our unconsciousness and become a natural part of our being.

To illustrate how affirmations work, let's look at eating apples. When we affirm "I am eating apples," we set into motion the changes necessary to eat an apple. In this case we may smell or taste the apple. We may feel the cool, firm apple in our hand or hear it crunch as our teeth bite into it. Our mind may focus on where we can get one and then our mind and body may take us to an apple and we'll find ourselves eating one. The thought creates the action.

When affirmations are used consistently, the body "learns" the action being affirmed. Experiments have been conducted in sports, particularly, with basketball players, that verified this phenomenon. Two players of relatively equal strength practiced for a week on their skills. One practiced on the court and the other practiced by visualizing the moves in his mind. When the players were put through a drill to retest their skills, the player who had used visualizations had improved slightly more than the person who practiced on the court. Experts believe that because the player using visualizations saw only success, he therefore, expected success, whereas the player on the court who made unsuccessful attempts had thoughts and pictures developed for those as well. Affirmations, and likewise visualizations, have a very powerful effect. When used consistently and with intention, affirmations can change our beliefs, which in turn will change our behaviors and outcomes.

Last January I coordinated an open house for the Agency for Hearing. We had moved into a new facility the previous fall. Originally we expected to have only about twenty people attending and to receive some free publicity. Six weeks before the event I created several affirmations and began repeating them every morning.

I use the power and authority of God to bring success.

In Your authority we provide a successful and memorable open house.

In Your authority we bring success and prosperity to the agency.

*Thank you, God, for gifting me with the mind,
energy, creativity, power, and will to bring success.*

*I allow Your energy to flow through me to manifest
this success. Success is what you expect me to
manifest.*

Somehow in six weeks I managed to find volunteers
to donate two large sheets of glass (to be used to "create
a noise" to get the attention of the community and
media), build a frame to hold the glass, find a volunteer
who designed and produced invitations at only the cost
of paper, and two volunteers who videotaped and shot
photos of the entire event. The publicity stunt attracted
more than one hundred people, including five politi-
cians and two television reporters, resulting in a two-
minute newsclip and one newspaper article featuring
our photo on the front page. Every morning when I read
over these affirmations I could feel my mind/body prepare for the day. I could feel my chest expand to take on
the challenges. I could feel myself focus on success. Affirmations changed my beliefs and therefore changed
the outcome making the event successful.

Affirmations are powerful.

To use affirmations to bring about positive change
in our life, we state or affirm what we want, even
though it may not appear to exist at the moment. We

may affirm, "I am a hearing Child of God," even though
we have a hearing loss. We affirm what we want as if it
exists. Spiritually it does exist, but it hasn't yet manifested itself to be visible in the body.

Sometimes using affirmations may make us feel
uncomfortable. How can we declare something to exist
when no physical evidence confirms that it does? How
can I say I am eating an apple, when one doesn't exist in
my hand? Having had success with changes, whenever
I feel my body or mind resist or feel uncomfortable, I
say to myself, "If it's uncomfortable, it means something is happening and I'm closer to changing that be-
havior/belief." I bless the change and "know" I am
closer to my goal. On the other hand, if the affirmations
bring up a violent reaction or I become physically ill
(both responses are rare, but they do happen occasionally) I decide it is better for me to move more slowly toward the change. Before I state the affirmation, I use the
phrase, "I am willing to consider. . . ." Using this phrase
gives me distance between my current belief and the
new belief I want to demonstrate. "I am willing to consider. . . . I am a hearing Child of God." "I am willing to
consider. . . . I communicate with ease." Using the
phrase "I am willing to consider" keeps me moving for-
ward toward my new belief while my body/mind ad-
justs to the different thinking pattern. My experience
has been that it works best to use the phrase "I am will-

ing to consider. . . ." for one or two weeks until I become comfortable making the affirmation without the phrase.

"I am" calls forth the power in the moment. At some point we may be tempted to use the phrases "I will be" or "I will have." When these phrases are used, what we call forth will remain in the future. We will always "be ready" to eat, but we may never eat an apple. The statement "I will eat apples" tells our body/mind we will eat apples at some point in the future. The statement "I am eating apples" tells our body/mind that right now, in the present moment, "I am eating apples." The body responds to what it can do now.

We will have better results if we use affirmations at a regular time. They might be part of our daily meditation time. Some people use them first thing in the morning to set the tone for the day. Some people use them before bedtime to calm themselves and give their mind an intention to work on while they sleep. Many do both. As we become more comfortable with using them, we often will re-affirm them throughout the day as needed. When I find myself losing focus or when I allow someone to distract me from my goals, I take a few moments of quiet time, preferably alone and outside in nature, to call forth my intent and reset my mind.

When I approach a new selection of affirmations or prayers to use, I like to read them over and select those that resonate with me or move me. Also, before using them on a regular basis, I like to establish an intent in my mind. I focus my energies on the change I want to occur. In my own words, I may say to myself, "I am open and receptive to new beliefs and I allow them in." Or, I may say to myself, "I want to release my (past, confusion, fear, pain) and allow God's good to guide my life."

When I start using a new affirmation, I often just repeat it in concentration. I consciously speak it to myself. As I get closer to shifting the new belief to the unconscious level, my intent becomes more focused. It has to, for I often feel that the old beliefs are screaming inside me and to continue the affirmations, I must focus with purpose. For me, the stronger I make the intent and the more I focus all my energies on it, the better the results.

What I mean by screaming is that it feels as if the more I affirm a new belief into my awareness, the more the old one seems to make me aware of its presence. Sometimes it seems to be screaming in my head, or numbing my thinking and feelings. Many users of affirmations say old beliefs resist change and fight for their life before they let go. However, I now have a different interpretation of the screaming and numbing I sometimes sense in my body. Last year I was using affirmations to call forth a change in my beliefs and was just starting to experience resistance when I felt a wave of relaxation pass through me. Instantly it became clear to me that the old belief wasn't fighting to stay alive at all. I saw that I merely interpreted the sensations as fighting. I understood with clarity that the old belief was just passing through my awareness while it was chemically breaking down to move out of my body. Dumbfounded, my years of believing old beliefs were fighting passed before me. I felt that belief collapse and quietly leave my body. The fight was gone. From then on I have had to be careful to release the habit of thinking old beliefs put up a fight. I use visualization to imagine in my mind a stubborn, large, old belief slowly breaking down and sense it is like watching a large clump of soil slowly breaking down into smaller clumps and eventually into fine particles that disappear from my awareness. And I imagine these belief clumps passing through my body with no intent to fight. Their usefulness in maintaining that old belief is no longer needed to support me; it is just evolving into another form to be useful elsewhere in the universe. It's just moving on. Now when I hear screaming or feel a numbing, I visualize a larger "clump" leaving the room through a keyhole where it tries to squeeze through the small hole. The "fight," if I want to interpret it that way, is the clump as it breaks down and leaves.

For me this is a much less stressful image of what is happening inside me when I go through a change. It also gives me the responsibility to further release the habit of the old belief. I see now it was I who was fighting to hold on to the belief, not the belief fighting to hold on to its existence. The power of releasing the old belief is within me.

I have a vivid internal visualization process and one of the patterns I use when working with a new affirmation is to imagine it as light and to imagine it in my mind. Then I repeat it while imagining it in my heart. Then I repeat it again while imagining it traveling to every cell in my body. I invite the new behavior or belief to enter into every cell in my body. I see it/feel it take hold in every cell. I breathe into my belly and allow the new pattern to become me. I imagine the affirmation forming a new path in my mind/body. With each repetition, I imagine the path deepening.

Science has shown that when we learn a new skill, form a new thought, or develop a new belief, we create chemical pathways in our mind/body. At first, the path is very thin. As we repeat the new skill, thought or belief, the path is reinforced. Eventually we develop a thick path and the new skill, thought, or belief becomes automatic and is done without thinking. For instance, when we learned to drive, it may have been difficult to judge how to move the car into a center lane to turn left. Now, after years of driving, that skill is now in our subconscious and we do it without much conscious thought.

Using affirmations develops and reinforces new chemical paths in the mind/body. With continued use, the paths become permanent. The old paths we no longer use begin to dissolve and fade away. As we affirm "I am a hearing Child of God," its path becomes stronger while any paths we have told our body, such as "nobody will want to accommodate you" or "you've got one foot in the grave," will start to dissolve, just as a path across a vacant lot will eventually disappear when a fence is installed.

I've used affirmations for years and now I can often feel my body respond to the words. I remember a pivotal experience in my belief of affirmations. I was preparing for a job interview. On a sample list of job interview questions, I had written the affirmation, "I am practiced and prepared for an interview." To prepare for an upcoming job interview I reviewed the list and as I read the affirmation I vividly remember my body moving me. I felt my posture straighten and my mind focus on the questions. I felt a shift inside. I felt power course through me. My intent zeroed in on getting that job. The power I felt from the affirmation startled me. I felt I had set into motion my preparedness for that job interview. From that moment on, I understood on a body level the power of words.

HOW SOON WILL I RECEIVE RESULTS?
AREN'T I SETTING MYSELF UP TO FAIL?

How soon we bring about changes through using affirmations depends on our belief in them, on how much the old beliefs mean to us, and on how ready we are to release these old beliefs.

How ready are we to consider that our words produce our outcomes? And positive words produce positive outcomes?

How ready are we to hold a picture of health in our mind?

How ready are we to release feeling isolated from others?

I find that the more I believe in God, the more I turn over to God, the less I feel I have to control every aspect of my life and the quicker—and easier—changes occur. Attempting to control everything leads me to hovering over every detail of my life. A new plant can't grow if I pull it up to measure its roots every two days. Hovering over every detail keeps me focused on the old details, the ones I want to release, so ultimately I'm reinforcing the old belief. We have to learn to trust or have faith that the changes will occur. We have to learn to expect the change, look for progress toward the change and celebrate even the tiniest improvement.

I remember many years ago I was so critical of every detail of my life I would emotionally beat myself up for all the "wrong" things I did. I was very judgmental. I was not only critical of what I did wrong, but I was critical of when I noticed I had done wrong. I judged myself bad for making a mistake and I judged myself bad for taking two months to realize I made a mistake. I was one "bad"—

misjudged—person. Then one day something different happened. I noticed a "wrong" action within a week after its occurrence, instead of the usual two months. I felt a wave of joy sweep through my body. I felt amazed at my success. Although the change was not in the behavior I observed, but only in when I noticed the behavior, it was a shift in my thinking. From that moment on I knew I could change. Intuitively I began to affirm "I celebrate all small changes." I looked for them. Soon I began to notice and celebrate those tiniest changes.

How soon we can bring about results may depend on how observant we are of the tiny changes that lead to the larger ones. Can we observe minute changes in our experience? Can we use the celebratory energy to further empower ourselves to create more positive results? The answer is yes, if we believe we can. We can listen. We can observe. We can open ourselves to shifts in our experience. How soon we bring about results depends on how soon we choose to notice them.

When we observe only big results, we remain disappointed. Disappointment indicates we are focusing on what we *don't* have; celebration indicates we are focusing on what we *do* have. We can choose to remain disappointed, or we can choose to celebrate. Which sounds like a better use of our energy and attention?

Sometimes the big results we want are not big enough. Recall the railroad trains of the 1800's for example. These monolithic beasts could travel from coast to coast in days, versus the months it took in covered wagons. But as automobiles and planes developed, the railroad industry eroded. Had railroad owners focused on the benefit they brought to their customers (i.e., transportation), they would have invested their profits in diversified forms of transportation and continued to experience success. In a similar way, when we focus on our hearing loss, we forget to focus on the benefits hearing brought us: communicating and feeling connected with others. Is it the hearing we want back, or do we want to feel connected with others?

We are whole beings. Just because one part of us (our hearing) is not functioning completely does not mean we can't communicate with others. Our experience will be different. We may be frustrated as we release dependence on one method of communicating and develop different methods to feel connected with others. We were comfortable with using hearing to feel connected; now we need to create new ways. We may employ existing, perhaps underdeveloped methods, such as being more observant of body language. We may find new methods, such as using lip reading and/or email.

Or we may invite God to help us discover alternatives outside our current awareness. Just as the railroad companies were blind to being in the transportation business, we may be blind to ways in which we can connect with others. We must open ourselves to different ways to get our needs met.

Being open may bring about unexplainable results. My mother's hearing loss rides on the bottom of the audiogram. In one ear her eardrum does not vibrate and her anvil, hammer and stirrup bones are fused together. Medically, doctors tell her she is deaf, yet she can hear in that ear. Doctors have no explanation for it, but have observed this phenomenon to occur in some people. Is it faith? Did she overcome physical limitations because she wanted to be connected with the world? I don't know. In this regard I'm glad my mother did not know the extent of her hearing loss, for if she had believed the doctors and viewed herself as deaf, she probably wouldn't hear as much as she can now. What you believe is more important than what others believe.

CAN AFFIRMATIONS REALLY BRING ABOUT PHYSICAL CHANGE?

I absolutely believe that the words we use and beliefs we hold result in changes in the body. When I watch someone's face change from rosy color to ashen when they are told a loved one has passed on, I know that words change the body. When a person with multiple personalities has a scar on his/her arm while in one personality and that scar is gone while he/she is in another personality, I know beliefs change the body. In my youth, while I was sitting next to my father in the car, he would squeeze my left knee in play. This hurt me. When I started dating I remember more than once when a guy went to set his hand on my leg my hand would lock his wrist inches above my leg. I was as surprised as anyone the first time it happened. As an adult I always had knee problems; I couldn't play catcher in softball because my left knee would give out. I always intuitivly believed I could heal the knee if I wanted to. And one day I did just that. I focused all my energies on my knee, reciting affirmations over and over. I visualized the pain released and gone forever. Eventually the pain harbored in my left knee disappeared. This experience and others have shown me that beliefs can manifest problems in our body, and that changing beliefs through the use of affirmations can remove or heal the problems. These ideas remained my private observations until I began studying metaphysical thought and began reading of people who had physical healings.

WHAT DOES THE STUDY OF METAPHYSICS SAY?

Physics shows we are energy fields represented as a moving mass of molecules, nuclei and atoms. Because we are in constant motion we can change our physical appearance. Our appearance changes when external actions happen to us: when we color our hair, have plastic surgery, or are burned in a fire. Our appearance can also change when internal things happen to us, such as a change of belief. Many people have reported physical healings after they have replaced thoughts of disease with thoughts of wholeness. Norman Cousins used humor to heal himself and others. He writes, "The greatest force in the human body is the natural drive of the body to heal itself—but that force is not independent of the belief system. . . . Everything begins with belief. What we believe is the most powerful option of all. . . ."

Metaphysically, how do we heal? How does the body heal a broken leg? Our bodies are made of energy. What we perceive as solid is in reality energy. Because our bodies are moving energy, energy cells can realign and become whole again. When we go to the doctor with a broken bone, all the doctor does is "set" the bone; our body does the healing. Cells in our body replace themselves every two years. Literally every two years we become a new person.

Damaged sensory hairs in the inner ear cochlea are the cause of hearing loss in the majority of those with hearing loss. Damage is attributed to exposure to loud noises, birth defects, diseases, and aging. Over the past decade, scientists have observed sensory hair cells growing in sharks and birds, and have successfully regenerated sensory hairs in guinea pigs. Excited to bring about cell regeneration of sensory hairs in humans, they continue their research. However, I believe we already have the power to regenerate sensory hairs and restore hearing. I believe that bones can heal so it is easy for me to imagine that parts in the ears can heal as well.

> "The time will come when the work of the physician will not be to treat and attempt to heal the body, but to heal the mind, which in turn will heal the body. The true physician will be a teacher. . . ."
>
> —RALPH W. TRINE

Physics shows that a thought can manifest material items. Take, for instance, the airplane. Watching a bird fly probably gave someone the idea that humans could fly. At that point it was only an idea. However, the idea led to thousands of experiments and eventually Wilbur and Orville Wright succeeded in flying. The original idea that man could fly resulted in a plane, a material item.

We all know people who have a poor attitude and never have things work out the way they say they desire. They say they want "ABC," yet they talk about what they won't get and how it won't work. It's no surprise they don't get the "ABC" they said they want and they continue to receive what they talk about most. The universe provides that which we most believe.

Long known by mystics and spiritual teachers, we are capable of healing ourselves. As Paul advised the

Romans, "Be ye transformed by the renewing of your mind." (Romans 12:2) We've read dozens of stories of people who have overcome cancer and lived twenty additional years or people with various diseases or injuries who recovered as a result of prayer. To the medical community, these healings are pronounced "miracles." To the spiritual community, these "miracles" are expected.

My spiritual beliefs are that we are all born spiritually perfect. I believe God is everywhere; therefore God is in us. If God is in us, then we are perfect, as is God. We are born feeling connected and at one with God. I've spoken with toddlers about God and have received vivid discussions of their experiences communicating with God. Small children seem to be in touch with God and speak of God with great familiarity. Unfortunately, by the time a child reaches five or seven, the open communication with God disappears. Unsupported by their earth experience, the connection fades away from their consciousness. They lose touch with God. Losing this sense of connection with God, we learn to believe we are separate beings. Invisible, our spiritual self is not well supported. When we cried as infants, we were told to be quiet. Yet crying was one of the only ways we could communicate our needs. We soon learned something was wrong with crying—with communicating our needs—and we learned to ignore our needs. The more

we learn to live in our earth world, the less we live in our
Spirit world. Eventually our earth-learned experience
and thoughts take over. We forget we are one with God.
We forget we are perfect, whole, and able to heal. The
part of us that we were taught to believe is imperfect *becomes* imperfect, and often mental, emotional or physical illnesses manifest and become a permanent part of
our experience. Too often we're taught to look outside of
us for the cause of an illness and to chase after remedies
and cures, when the answers exist within us.

Since we sometimes stray from our spiritual awareness that we are one with all, we receive signals (i.e.,
emotions such as anger or pain) alerting us we have
strayed. But if we ignore them or have forgotten what
they mean, the unexpressed energy remains in our body.
Unused, unexpressed energy eventually manifests into
some physical condition. As we return to our original
spiritual belief that we are one with God and we listen to
the signals we receive, the energy flows again and the
physical condition created disappears. This is how we
heal. For some this happens in an instant. For most it
happens slowly.

As we grow older and continue to not listen to and
not act upon body messages we receive, we often encounter cancer, heart attacks, or major accidents or illnesses that encourage us to get back in touch with our
spiritual self. For some, hearing loss is that opportunity.

WHAT DO HEALERS AND
OTHERS WITH EXPERIENCE SAY?

In studies, books and on the Internet are hundreds of accounts of people healing themselves through prayer and affirmations. Writer and publisher Louise Hay healed herself of cancer using prayers and affirmations. Drawing upon ancient healing practices from around the world, she later wrote the book *You Can Heal Your Life*, in which she lists dozens of physical conditions. She identifies beliefs or thinking patterns that tend to manifest each specific condition and suggests an affirmation that will help release the belief or thinking pattern.

When I was introduced to her work more than fifteen years ago I intuitively recognized that she was right. At the time I recalled the marriage I postponed when I awakened the morning of the wedding physically unable to get out of bed. Before I became ill, I "knew" the marriage wouldn't last more than two months, but I couldn't say no. My body helped me. Three days later I cancelled the wedding altogether. I had to become physically ill before I listened to myself.

I use Hay's book now whenever I have a physical condition that suddenly appears. I'll look up the physical condition and see what thinking pattern is associated with it. If her analysis resonates with my experience, I'll write down the affirmation and begin using it. If it doesn't resonate with my experience, I disregard it and focus on listening to my body for other clues. More than 80% of the time the thinking pattern is exactly what's going on in my mind. We don't always want to hear that something we believe is causing a physical condition. We're more comfortable thinking it's just something that happened to us or blaming someone or something else. We're also more comfortable going to a doctor and expecting a medical treatment to fix it. But we have the power to heal our illnesses and injuries.

In the book, *Tapping the Healer Within*, author Roger J. Callahan explains a system he developed of finger tapping and eye movements to release the emotional blocks and psychological problems that prevent us from fully living our lives. He relates stories of sessions lasting ten minutes where tapping removed phobias in dozens of people. One woman with a phobia of water could not get near it. She could not take a bath and could barely take a quick shower feeling terror the entire time she did. Roger took her through the tapping system and she immediately went to the pool and splashed water in her face. He's also had positive results with physical healings. Callahan, well studied in applied kinesiology, acupuncture, neurolinguistic programming and various quantum theories, discovered the technique intuitively. He listened to his intuition, God, Spirit,—whatever we want to call it—and discovered a healing method we can all use. I've read and experienced other methods of healing that have been developed recently, as well as ancient methods. Our Western culture is accepting more belief-based natural healings, rather than relying exclusively on intrusive, external methods of fixing or replacing.

IS THERE A CONNECTION BETWEEN MY BELIEFS AND MY HEARING LOSS?

Many metaphysical healers are certain that what we believe reflects in our physical expression. In her book, Louise Hay does not specifically address hearing loss, but gives what ears represent generally. For each physical condition she gives a probable cause (a thought or belief) and a new thought pattern we can use to release the old beliefs no longer working for us. On the following page is what her studies have revealed about ears, earache, deafness and tinnitus:

My mother lost her hearing at the age of five when she had an ear infection, which today would have been cleared up with antibiotics. But her home life was not harmonious; there was fighting in her household. Plus, she had always felt her father didn't love her. I concluded she did not like what she was hearing and manifested the ear infection. Unable to hear, she could not hear the tur-

EAR(S)

Probable Cause
Represents the capacity to hear.

New Thought Pattern
I hear with love.

EARACHE

Probable Cause
Anger. Not wanting to hear. Too much turmoil.
Parents arguing.

New Thought Pattern
Harmony surrounds me. I listen with love to the pleasant
and the good. I am a center for love.

DEAFNESS

Probable Cause
Rejection, stubbornness, isolation. What don't you want
to hear? "Don't bother me."

New Thought Pattern
I listen to the Divine and rejoice at all that I am able to
hear. I am one with all.

TINNITUS

Probable Cause
Refusal to listen. Not hearing the inner voice.
Stubbornness.

New Thought Pattern
I trust my Higher Self. I listen with love to my inner voice.
I release all that is unlike the action of love.

moil and anger in her home. Also, a hearing loss gave her a reason why she never heard "I love you" from her father.

But, I asked myself, what about those of us who lose our hearing when we are older? Could it be we are angry at what we hear around us? Could it be we do not want to hear what is being said? Could it be we feel we have too much turmoil and want to leave it behind? Could it be our parents are still arguing in our head after forty or fifty years and we want to shut them out? Could it be we feel we've lost our power or our source of recognition (especially after retirement)? Could it be we have lost touch with our inner voice, our sense of connection with God? If we seem to resonate with any of these ideas, we may choose to meditate on them to understand them more deeply for our personal situation. And/or we may use the affirmations given—or create our own—to change our thinking.

Working on the spiritual level takes belief and consistent practice. Practicing prayers and affirmations daily will improve our ability to listen to our body. In addition to meditating on the affirmations, we might focus on our ears. We can ask them what we can do to increase our hearing. In meditation, we can also see them healthy, whole and healed. If we resonate with any of Hay's probable causes, we can ask our ears what lesson we need to learn to restore our hearing. Consider what new thought patterns we may need to adopt—

or, more likely, we were trained as children to forget. God knows the answer. I believe our body knows the answer. The answers are there when we listen.

God, what lesson am I to learn to restore my hearing?

I am willing to learn that lesson now.

I see my ears healthy, whole and fully functioning.

I am a hearing child of God.

PHYSICAL HEALINGS FROM PRAYERS

Myrtle Fillmore, who later became one of the co-founders of Unity, had always been a sickly child. In her mid-forties she was told by doctors that she would not live another six months, having at the time what they called "consumption." Myrtle had been studying New Thought ideas and when told the doctor's prediction, she fervently continued her search. At a lecture she heard the words, "You are a child of God and do not inherit sickness." This idea resonated with her and she began prayers. She prayed and affirmed she was a child of God. She affirmed she did not inherit sickness and it was not part of her being. She imagined herself as whole and well.

In her pamphlet, *How I Found Health* she wrote:

Life is simply a form of energy, and has to be guided and directed in man's body by his intelligence. How do we communicate with intelligence? By thinking and talking, of course.

Then it flashed upon me that I might talk to the life in every part of my body and have it do just what I wanted. I began to teach my body and got marvelous results.

I told the life in my liver that I was not torpid or inert, but full of vigor and energy. I told the life in my stomach that it was not weak or inefficient, but energetic, strong, and intelligent. I told the life in my abdomen that it was no longer infested with ignorant thoughts of disease . . . but that it was all a thrill with the sweet, pure, wholesome energy of God. I told my limbs that they were active and strong.

I went to all the life centers in my body and spoke words of Truth to them—words of strength and power. I asked their forgiveness for the foolish, ignorant course that I had pursued in the past when I had condemned them and called them weak, inefficient, and diseased. I did not become discouraged at their being slow to wake up, but kept right on, both silently and aloud, declaring the words of Truth, until the organs responded."

At the end of two years Myrtle no longer had consumption, nor was sickly, as before. She went on to live for another forty-five active years.

After her healing, her husband, Charles, began using prayers to heal a lifetime hip disease that affected the whole right side of his body, including deafness in his right ear. In his book, *Atom Smashing Power of Mind* he wrote:

> I can testify to my own healing of tuberculosis of the hip. When a boy of ten I was taken with what was at first diagnosed as rheumatism, but developed into a very serious case of hip disease. I was in bed over a year, and from that time on I was an invalid in constant pain for twenty-five years.
>
> Two tubercular abscesses developed at the head of the hip bone. I managed to get about on crutches, with a four-inch cork-and-steel extension on the right leg. The hip bone was out of the socket and stiff. The leg shriveled and ceased to grow. The whole right side became involved; my right ear was deaf and my right eye weak.
>
> When I began applying the spiritual treatment there was for a long time slight response in the leg, but I felt better, and I found that I began to hear with the right ear. Then gradually I noticed that I had more feeling in the leg . . . the ossified joint began to get limber . . . the shrunken flesh filled out until the right leg was al-

most equal to the other . . . I . . . wore an ordinary shoe with a double heel about an inch in height.

I have watched the restoration . . . as I applied the power of thought, and I know it is under divine law. So I am satisfied that here is proof of a law that the mind builds the body and can restore it.

I believe we can manifest a complete healing of hearing loss, but we will need discipline and belief to manifest a complete physical change. It is not something completed on a Sunday afternoon. Some believe it is possible in one session, as happened in the case of the healings Jesus performed, but, more likely, it may take several weeks or months of concentrated effort for a change in our current belief system to manifest a physical change. However, I believe most of us will improve the experience of hearing loss by using prayers and affirmations.

Improvements may come in different forms. Opening our mind and heart to the possibility that a physical healing can happen opens our mind and heart to accept improvements. After several sessions with affirmations, we may be more inclined to take a lip reading class to enhance our reception of what others are saying. We may be more inclined to share hearing-related frustrations with others and speak our feelings. By releasing some of our anger we may shift into seeing the humor in difficult situations. Seeing the humor will lighten up our perspective and the world may not seem so dark and unforgiving.

All healing doesn't have to be manifested by our thought alone. Affirmations may open us to the possibility that other people or other equipment can help improve our hearing. Affirmations may give us the courage to speak up to request that others slow down their speech and speak clearly. Affirmations may open us to exploring stronger hearing aids or other assistive listening devices to improve communication. Affirmations may open us to the possibility of risking surgery that could improve our hearing. God works in mysterious ways.

A chiropractor friend of mind reports that she has had cases of people improving their hearing through chiropractic care. She shared with me that the first chiropractic session performed by Dr. Palmer, the founder of chiropractic care in the United States, improved a man's hearing. The man's back had been injured and he had also lost his hearing. Treatments were performed, the man's back healed, and his hearing was restored.

Science now shows that in the spinal column the hearing nerves are on the outside of the bundle of nerves against the bones. When bones are jarred out of place, the hearing nerves can be restricted or damaged. Apparently, in this case, the chiropractic adjustment shifted the bones to release the pressure against the hearing nerves and his hearing was restored. I've heard of similar healings of hearing loss resulting from using foot reflexology. We never know where or how improvements can be made, but they do occur.

As we allow ourselves to be open and receptive to listening—to God, to our body, to our heart—we are directed to what will bring us improvement.

I am open and receptive to God's guidance.

I am willing to consider I may improve my hearing.

I am willing to consider I am a hearing child of God.

3

How Do I Begin?

All of us use affirmations whether we realize it or not. Most of us used them when we learned to ride a bike, drive a car, or memorize multiplication tables. We probably repeated something like, "I can do it. I can learn this." We may not have called them affirmations, but most of us reassured ourselves that we could perform the new task.

Whether we're drawing upon our personal faith or have used affirmations before, we first need to believe they can work and be open to see what positive changes we can have. Our success with affirmations is determined by our belief and the commitment we give to staying focused on the positive outcomes.

Using affirmations consistently will change our beliefs about hearing loss, keep us positive during those moments of frustration, and reinforce our decision to find success in spite of the loss. (Some of us may have to pretend to believe, until we see or feel improvements.)

*I am open and receptive to a change in my hearing
loss experience.*

*I am willing to accept into my life the benefits a
hearing loss can bring me.*

*I am ready to heal; I am ready to improve my
hearing loss experience.*

CREATING A POSITIVE IMAGE OF OURSELVES

It's amazing how our beliefs shape us. Some of us, when we admit we have a hearing loss became "older" overnight, for we've been thinking anyone with a hearing loss has "one foot in the grave" or is "one step away from death." But these beliefs are not true. If we find ourselves with "negative" associations about hearing loss, we can ask ourselves, "Are they real or are they imagined?" Then we can create positive images of ourselves with a hearing loss. We can see ourselves with a bounce in our step, we can see ourselves with bright, clear face color and we can see ourselves active and interested in life. Any old, untrue beliefs we hold will dissolve when we re-train our mind with positive images.

With improved hearing aid technology many of us will make minor modifications to our current activities. Hearing aids are now less visible, more powerful and more effective than they were in the past. They are becoming common and no longer a stigma.

Since the inception of ADA (Americans with Disabilities Act), society is more accepting of people who have disabilities and more open to making accommodations. When we ask for accommodations with confidence and expect we'll receive them, we dramatically increase our success. Today, many of us with hearing loss seem to blend in with others. We train those in our lives what we require to participate in life and find the courage to regularly remind them to speak up and speak clearly. Affirmations develop and support a proactive image and attitude in which we can achieve success with hearing loss.

I am alive, active and live with a bounce in my step.

I solve challenges with ease and confidence.

I boldly ask others to accommodate my loss to help me remain connected.

DEVELOPING OUR "THIRD EAR"

If we were to become blind, our sense of hearing becomes more acute. Likewise, if we were to lose our hearing, our other senses would become sharper. As we open

ourselves to the possibilities of communicating through
these other channels we develop our "third ear." Reading
body language, paying attention to scents, being observant to the heat or coolness on our skin, we will soon
seem to be able to "sense" another person speaking. We
can become highly sensitive to olfactory signals and notice from a scent that some person has entered the room.
We can be more aware of communication clues such as
blushing, gestures, or posture. According to experts,
50% of communication that is shared with another is
transmitted by our body language and visual cues. Most
of us are not consciously aware we use visual cues, but
the look in an eye or the shrug of a shoulder visually sup-
ports what we verbally communicate. Practice in observing will produce results quickly. Turn the sound down on
your favorite television sitcom and see how much of the
story you can follow. Go to a public place and observe a
conversation: what do you think they are talking about?
How do they feel about the subject (even if you aren't
aware of the subject matter)? Many of us do not think we
can learn lip reading, but when we give ourselves permission to take a class we find out in the first session
how much we already use lip reading—and we didn't
even know it. Some, by the way, refer to it as Speech
Reading, broadening their ability to read clues from the
whole body, the whole message being sent, not just from
reading lips. With practice we can develop the use of intuition, our sixth sense. The purpose here is to open our-

selves to the signals sent. As children we knew them well; most of us have gotten out of the habit of consciously using them. Any additional ideas of ways to develop our "third ear" should be tried. Developing our third ear will decrease our communication frustrations and increase our communication success.

My third ear hears clearly and with confidence.

I read body language and visual cues with ease.

My senses are sharp; I know what's going on around me.

I lip read with ease.

BUILDING UP OUR RESERVES FOR THE LONG HAUL

One of the greatest frustrations of hearing loss is to continually ask for accommodations. "Can you speak up?" "What did you say?" "Can you face me when you speak?" It slows down communications and wears us out. Many of us feel it's easier not to deal with the constant inconvenience but then we soon find ourselves isolated from others. Not wanting to remain isolated, we boldly venture out among people again. We can use affirmations throughout our day to recharge ourselves so we can continue to advocate when we cannot understand. We can fortify ourselves with affirmations before we place a call to a hotel to request hearing accommodations, or before we go shopping and have to ask the store clerk to speak up, or before we meet with friends and have to continually remind them to face us when speaking. When we use affirmations regularly we can keep fueled and energized to stay positive and to expect success in encounters with others. Along with fortifying ourselves with affirmations, we also need to thank everyone who accommodates us. Gratitude encourages others to continue supporting us and acknowledging others who understand our needs keeps us energized as well.

I effortlessly remind others to look at me.

I bless those who look at me and speak clearly.

I am connected with those around me.

I am successful in all my communications.

WRITING OUR OWN AFFIRMATIONS

We can write our own affirmations for any situation. We can write affirmations for upcoming surgery to affirm success with the surgery and also with our communications with hospital staff. We can plan how best we can accommodate ourselves at a large family gathering and create affirmations that affirm a positive, relaxing outcome. We can create affirmations when we take a class to call forth an understanding and accommodating instructor.

The more specific we make them, the more powerful they can be. Follow these guidelines when making affirmations:

- Keep the language in present tense (I am, we are, it is, etc.).

- Affirm what you want (this may be a challenge at first for we're so used to identifying what we don't want).

- Use simple statements such that a five-year-old could understand them. Simple sentences are readily understood by the subconscious.

After using affirmations from this book, writing your own affirmations will become easy. It may be a struggle at first to make them positive as our society is so used to thinking with negative thought patterns, but keep at it. Following are some affirmations addressing issues discussed in this section.

I write affirmations with ease.

I am calm and relaxed for tomorrow's successful surgery.

I bless the doctor and attendants for their skills and talents.

I am relaxed with my family. I am creative in understanding my family.

I am blessed with an enriching experience.

I understand the instructor with clarity and ease.

I see accommodations used with ease in my classroom.

I am filled with joy and peace in the classroom.

4

Hearing Affirmations

ffirmations are helpful tools that guide us toward our goals and desires. As you recall in Chapter 2, we discussed the affirmation process and how it works. Before you read this chapter, it might be helpful to review these key points.

- Affirmations identify what we want in our life.

- Affirmations prepare our mind for the outcome we expect.

- Affirmations are written in the present tense.

- Affirmations must be spoken out loud, thought "out loud" in your mind, or written.

- Affirmations are powerful when used consistently with intention.

As you read these affirmations, be very deliberate, taking your time to fully understand every word before deciding which are best suited for you. It's my sincere hope that you discover certain affirmations that resonate with your situation and desire.

Be ye transformed by the renewing of your mind.
—ROMANS 12:2

I Am Alive with Energy

Life, a healing, restorative energy, courses
through my body, mind, and soul.

I am alive and I feel God's life energy
awaken my cells, awaken my dreams, and
awaken my being to call me forth.

I have more life to experience.

I have more to give.

I have more to receive.

I have more to hear.

I feel God's life energy healing my ears,
restoring life to the nerve endings,
the bones, the cochlea and all parts of the ear,
nerves and mind that help me hear.

I hear with the clarity of a healthy newborn baby.

Thank you, God, for returning to me my hearing.

I appreciate each word said to me.

I am alive with energy.

I Am a Hearing Child of God

I am a child of God and I do not inherit illness.

I am complete, whole and a perfect expression of God.

I am open to the joy and love that surround me.

I hear the joy and love expressing abundantly
in my life.

I bless my hearing.

I bless my ears.

I bless my middle ear.

I bless my inner ear.

I bless my ear canal.

I bless my eardrum.

I bless my inner ear canal.

I bless my anvil, stirrup and hammer bones.

I bless my inner ear fluids.

I bless my inner ear nerve endings.

I bless the nerves that transmit the
flow of the fluids to my brain.

I bless my brain, which interprets
the sound waves into words.

I bless my mind, which sees each word
as an expression of love.

I bless my heart, which welcomes all
expressions of love into my life.

I bless my body, which enjoys the stimulation of
those expressions of love.

I bless my soul, which thrives on
those expressions of love.

I bless my perfect hearing, which brings me
all these joys in my life.

Thank you God, for all that you have given me.

I am blessed.

I Welcome Every Word

I hear clearly each sound around me.

I welcome each word into my experience,
for words represent life—my life.

Each word said to me is my experience and
I cherish each word for it enriches
my understanding and
provides me opportunities to grow and
learn more about myself.

Thank you, God, for enriching my life.

I welcome every word.

Words Connect Me with Everyone

Words are the bridges on which relationships are built.

Words are the vehicles that transport love and
joy between souls.

Words bathe me in the bliss and blessings of others.

Words lead me to my inner peace.

I hear each word spoken to me.

I hear each word connecting me to others.

I hear each word bridging my relationships
to those in my life.

I hear each word transporting
love and joy to my soul.

I hear each word that bathes me in the bliss and
the blessings of others.

I hear each word that brings me peace.

I am open and receptive to the
spoken words in my life.

Thank you, God, for connecting me with words.

I connect with everyone.

Divine Life Lives In Me

Divine life lives in my body, mind, and soul.

Divine life awakens me to the joys of living.

Divine life enhances my life experience.

I hear the many blessings in my life.

I feel the many joys.

I am in wonder at the many ways
love expresses in my life.

Divine life calls me forth
to the lessons I am to learn.

Divine life calls me forth
to the abundance awaiting me.

Divine life calls me forth
to fulfill my purpose on earth.

I hear the many words God sends to support me.

I hear the many words God has for love expressing.

I hear all the words God means for me to hear.

Divine life sharpens my hearing.

I hear clearly.

Thank you, God.

I hear God's every message and every blessing.

The Healing Spirit Is At Work

The healing life of Spirit restores hearing to my ears.

Spirit moves through me quietly and
quickly to restore hearing to my life.

Spirit heals the cells in my ears,
my bones, my nerves, and my
mind to return to my life the
understanding of spoken words.

I hear all words.

I understand all words.

I hear clearly the messages sent to me.

I understand clearly the meaning of each word spoken.

I have healthy ears.

I have healthy hearing.

I am whole and complete.

Thank you, God, for giving me the healing Spirit.

The healing Spirit is at work.

I Am Forever Healing and Transforming

My body is continually changing.

Each moment of each day my body renews itself.

I replace discarded cells with life-filled,

newly energized cells charged with God's light.

I am a love-filled child of God.

Endowed with healing powers, I see myself healthy.

I am a hearing child of God.

My words call forth the renewing cells to
transform my wounds and renew my faith.

I am a hearing child of God.

Thank you, God, for the daily renewal of life.

I am forever healing and transforming.

I Am Grateful for My Silence

I am grateful for this hearing experience.

In the quiet I have grown to a deeper understanding
of myself and a greater appreciation of others.

I rest from the chaos around me.

I find peace and strength in the silence and appreciate
the time to reflect on life and on relationships.

Thank you, God, for allowing me to hear
exactly what I need to hear,
when I need to hear it,
and how I need to hear it.

I am grateful for my quiet and my peace.

I Am Learning a New Life Lesson

To broaden my life experience,
I am becoming acquainted with a new part of myself.
I am deepening my growth in other parts of myself.
I am learning patience.
I am learning acceptance.
I am learning forgiveness.
I am learning to move through frustration to joy.
I am challenging my sense of self-worth.
I am learning to ask for what I want.
I am learning how to let others help me.
I am learning to appreciate my resourcefulness.
I appreciate my creativity.
I am befriending my inner self.
I am learning to accept joy.
I am learning to appreciate self-love.
I am learning to find happiness in the moment.
I am willing to find new paths to happiness.
I am learning to connect with others in new ways.
Thank you, God, for this chance
to keep my life fresh and alive!

I am learning.

I Communicate On New Levels

I communicate with others on many levels.

In my temporary silence,
I experience more fully the levels
I have taken for granted.

I reach deeper into the depths of
my being for a richer experience of life.

Thank you, God, for I am grateful
for this opportunity.

I am communicating.

I Forgive Myself for
Believing I Cannot Hear

I have been given the necessary elements to hear
clearly. The elements in my ears and brain must all
work in harmony to receive sound and hear clearly.
My ears and brain are whole and complete.

Forgive me, ears,
for I believed you could not hear.
You can hear. I honor you, I appreciate you and
I see you as whole and serving me perfectly.

Forgive me, eardrum,
for I believed you
were not whole, healthy and vibrating freely.
You are complete.

Forgive me, inner ear nerves,
for I believed
you were not complete and capable of reading and
transmitting signals to my brain.
I hear and know the love of others.
You are capable.

Forgive me, cochlea,
for I believed you had
failed me. You are healthy and
transmitting sounds to my brain clearly.

Forgive me, brain,
for I believed you could
not interpret the signals sent from the nerves.
You interpret signals quickly and accurately.

Forgive me, ears,
for not taking better care of you.
I did not know. I now know.
I honor and care for my ears.

Ears, I am grateful that you connect me
with the world, with living, with life.

Ears, I am grateful that you connect me with
the joy and peace, blessing me each day.

Ears, I am grateful for the years of service
you have given me and you will continue to give me.

Thank you, God, for giving me all I need to hear.

I forgive myself for believing I cannot hear.

I hear clearly.

I Am Awakened to My Diverse, Power-filled Self

Certain traditions believe we possess twelve powers that have their energy centers in the body. When we call upon these powers, the spiritual, mental, and physical aspects of our being are more fully experienced and we come closer to reaching our higher (divine) potential. Following is an affirmation from each power center.

I am awakened to my diverse, power-filled self.

FAITH
In faith I believe I hear all.

STRENGTH
My strength through God makes me strong in mind, body, and spirit. My strength gives me courage to hear and to live my life fully.

WISDOM
I wisely allow in those words meant for me. I wisely screen out those words meant for others.

LOVE
I attract only loving words, people, and experiences into my life. I am immersed in abundant love, nurturing, calming and soothing every fiber of my being.

POWER
I am filled with God's power. With ease and confidence I receive others into my life.

IMAGINATION
I imagine and I am. Right now I am a healthy, loving,
hearing being filled with peace and joy.

UNDERSTANDING
My understanding is clear and aligned with Spirit.
I am a hearing child of God and full of love.

WILL
Aligned with God's will, I will myself into perfect
hearing health.

ORDER
Every cell in my body is in
divine order and I hear perfectly.

ZEAL
With zeal I expect perfect health at all times.
I am perfect health.

ELIMINATION
I release all "limiting hearing" thoughts from my
mind, body, and soul.

LIFE
Divine life moves in and through
every cell in my body. I hear perfectly.

Thank you, God.

I am grateful for the divine healing I have received.

Silence Is Golden

In the silence I experience another part of me,
one I have not taken the time before to know well.

Inside I find love streaming from my heart,
bringing peace and joy to every cell in my body.

I learn compassion for myself,
for the quiet parts of me that have sometimes been
overlooked.

I explore the hidden subtleties of my being
and honor their importance in my life.

Without the silence, I would not have known them.

This silence is golden.

Thank you, God.

I am aware of my unspoken essence.

I Attract Only Love

I attract only loving people,
loving words, loving thoughts, and
loving actions into my life.

Each moment of each day I am surrounded in love.

I hear love enter my body, mind, and
soul each day, and I rejoice.

The power of God helps me to release all that is
limited, false, and outworn obstructing my spiritual
unfoldment. I am free of limiting behaviors.

I am free to hear everyone in my life.

I am open and receptive to the sounds in my life.

I hear clearly everyone's love in expression.

I appreciate each sound, each tone,
even each noise in my life experience.

Words stimulate and enrich my life experience.

I hear each word clearly.

I allow in the joy of each spoken word.

Thank you, God for the eternal flow of
love throughout my life.

I attract only love.

I Am Blessed with Unspoken Words

I enrich my life through expressions of joy,
love, and peace, as well as expressions of
sorrow, grief, and pain.

All words, spoken or unspoken, enrich my experience
and make me complete.

I am blessed that I understand what others give me, for
they give more than words.

A look in their eye tells me more than words ever will.
A gesture of a hand or shoulder lets me know
what they are communicating. Their posture,
the color in their face, and their expression tell me
what I need to know. Their voice tone, pace, and
pitch communicate volumes. I only have to
"listen" to receive their message.

I open myself to the multiple messages
sent to me each day.

I open my heart to appreciate their subtleties and
experience their bliss.

Thank you, God, for the intuitive ability to
connect with others.

I am blessed with a fuller understanding and
appreciation of unspoken communications.

Love and Joy Fill My Life

Love and joy enter my ears,
stream through my mind and nerves, and
enter my heart instantly.
My ears are the doors to the love and
joys in my life. I open my ears to let in each and
every joy meant for me. I open my ears and
invite in the many expressions of love abundant
in my life. I open my ears and welcome the
words that connect me with everyone in my life.
I bless my ears, my doorways to others.

Thank you, God,
for all the ways love enters my life.

I am filled with love.

I Feel the Power of God

I feel God move in me as I hear all words of
living an abundant life.

I allow God to work through me and my ears.

God transforms my ears.

I claim my divine freedom to hear.

I am free to enjoy my life.

Thank you, God, for my divine freedom to hear.

I feel the power of God at work.

My Ears Are Open and Healthy

I am blessed with the richness of hearing every
expression of love and joy in my life.

My ears are open and healthy.
Words flow through my ear canals and
vibrate down my nerves,
transforming into meaning in my mind and
expressing themselves as love and
joy in my heart. I capture each word and
meaning meant for me.

I bathe in each word God sends my way.

Thank you, God.

I am a hearing child of God and I hear all.

The Joyful Spirit In Music

Music brings joy to my soul.

The spirit of music weaves itself into
my being and I am blessed.

I surround myself in a symphony of love.
Soothing string sounds lift me.

Winsome woodwind sounds fill me with breath.
Blaring brass sounds awaken my senses.
Penetrating percussion sounds reverberate
clearly into my heart and soul.

I hear in my mind and soul the
joyous symphony of music.

Sounds connect in my mind,
ripple through my soul, and fill me with
peace and joy.

My heart hears music and bursts to let me know
I am blessed. Blessings sweep my soul.

Delightful melodies awaken my mind and
inspire me to live for the moment.

Rhythms bounce me, staccatos move me, and
allegros soothe me as I float in delightful love.

I draw upon music in my heart,
savoring its subtle harmonies, melodies, and
feelings being expressed.

My soul "hears" the joys of songs. Sweet notes wash
over me, blessing me with gentle vibrations
that resonate and resound in my heart,
filling me with life.

I expand my experience of life
through new avenues, in ways that hadn't
occurred to me before but which the
universe provides me now.

I am open and receptive to God's experience.

I hear all sounds of love God shares with me.

I am fulfilled, loved, and satisfied.

I feel loved. I feel blessed.

Thank you, God, for the joyful spirit in music.

I am inspired by the
harmonious sounds of love filling my life.

The Essence of Nature Is Within Me

I am one with nature.

I feel the sun warm my face.
I feel breezes kiss my lips and I hear birds sing.

Above me, around me, they dance.
Calling to my soul I hear their gentle sweetness.

Babbling waters sing in my ears.

Wind-filled trees whisper in my heart.

Birds chirp sweet nothings.

The ocean pounds the shore and
dances blithely across the sands.

As I encounter nature, my ears, my mind,
heart, and soul are blessed.

I am one with nature and
I am one with sounds, as I am one with God.

All God experiences, I experience.

My third ear hears and blessings shower upon me.

Connected with nature in untold ways,
I feel at peace and
surrender limiting thoughts.

I open myself to the full experience of
God's creation and allow these blessings
to refresh my thoughts and my soul
just as rain cleanses the earth.

Thank you, God,
for allowing me to share in the wonder of nature.

I am one with nature as I am one with God.

I Experience Life Fully

I am willing to experience life fully.

I open my heart and mind to the
complete expression of life around me.

I am filled with love and joy,
and am happy to be alive.

Before now I was afraid to hear,
afraid of what others said they thought of me.

I was afraid of their anger and rage,
afraid of the pain I had felt in life.

I no longer hear those harmful words,
but now I have closed off all the words
of my life experience.

I am ready to hear all words again.

I know all people have a Spirit center within them
where pure love, joy, peace and safety reside.

This is their true self, their spiritual self.

Their true self is all good. It expresses only love.

It lives in joy and peace.

What others may say negative about me
comes not from their spiritual self but from
their own earth-learned behaviors.

Their anger and rage seemingly directed
toward me come from their own storehouse
of anger and rage built up over the years.
I may be this moment's target, but someone else or
something else will be their target in the
next moment.
It is not I with whom they are angry,
but some past deed they have not yet resolved.

The pain I have been afraid to feel
in my life is part of living.

I now know to comfort my pain,
to nurture my pain, and to surround my pain in love,

and the pain will be transformed and
released the moment I do.

My life is enriched with the experience of pain.
Hurts, angers, fears and pains received from others,
however, are not mine to keep.

I release all hurts, anger, fears, and
pain from my experience.

I forgive myself for believing they were mine to keep.

As they leave me, love fills in their void.

Love slips in to heal and to fill the space now empty.

(continued)

I Experience Life Fully, *(continued)*

I may experience some loss from
letting go of those familiar feelings, and
that is normal.
As I focus on the joy and love taking their place,
that feeling will heal, too.

I am a child of God, born without fears,
hurts, anger, or pain.

I have no need to hold on to them and
release them from my experience.

I am free of fears, hurts, anger and pain.
I am ready to hear words again.

I deflect other's anger, fears or hurts that
are falsely directed toward me.

Their misdirected words are not mine and
I do not let them enter my mind,
body, or soul. Rather, I have
compassion for those who would direct
such words at me in error.
I bless them and send them love
and healing thoughts.

Thank you, God, for giving life without
fear, hurt, anger, or pain.

I experience life fully.

CHAPTER 5

What Else Can I Do to Support My Hearing Loss?

M oving through the grieving process and using affirmations will eventually move you to take action. Many opportunities and resources are available to you as you become open to using them.

BOOKS

If you haven't already read a basic hearing loss book, I highly encourage you to do so. Understanding how the ear and mind work together will assist in healing your hearing loss through affirmations. Also you'll become empowered through understanding how and why your specific hearing loss exists. Knowledge is power. When the doctor explained your loss to you the first time, you were likely in shock and may recall little of what the doctor said. If you haven't done so already, read a basic hearing loss book to get more familiar with the process and terminology and then ask the doctor to explain you hearing loss again. Ask questions until you have a firm understanding. Bring a book with pictures if that helps you understand.

Preparing for a recent surgery, my mother was told by her doctor that her eardrum did not vibrate and let through sounds. It was the first time she had been told this during her sixty years of hearing loss. When she asked how she could hear, she was told that when sounds were loud enough they would circumvent the eardrum and cause vibrations in the middle ear anyway. This information helped her to understand just how loud sounds needed to be before she could hear them in that ear. Also, having that knowledge gave her an opportunity to create affirmations to soften or add flexibility to the eardrum. Understanding the specifics about your loss is important. When you meet with doctors, remember they will address the physical level of your hearing loss. Also remember that on a spiritual level hearing loss is not your true self.

Hearing loss books are rarely found in your local bookstore, but they can be ordered. Check with your public library for titles, and have the librarian check with the State Library if necessary. I was surprised to find that my local library system had six or seven books on hearing loss. If your library system does not have a basic book on hearing loss, ask that they get one. There are many excellent books. I'm listing a few suggested titles that I'm familiar with by topic that will provide a general introduction.

Books On Hearing Loss Basics

Living Well with Hearing Loss
by Debbie Huning

Coping with Hearing Loss
by Susan V. Rozen and Carl Hausman

Books On Hearing Loss Psychology & Insights

A Quiet World
by David Meyers

The Odyssey of Hearing Loss: Tales of Triumph
by Michael A. Harvey, Ph.D.

Books On Healing Affirmations

If you'd like additional reading on healing using affirmations, I suggest that you begin by reading Louise L. Hay's book, *You Can Heal Your Life*. Her book is a stimulating introduction to the concepts of affirmations and healings. I found two of Catherine Ponder's books, *The Dynamic Laws of Healing* and *The Healing Secrets of the Ages*, easy to read and helpful as well. You'll find other titles in your bookstore or library under the subject headings Metaphysical Studies, New Age, or New Thought.

INTERNET WEBSITES

If you or your family members are Internet savvy, there is much information available on the Internet. Most is medical related; however, there are sites that sell assistive listening devices, offer support, and cover legislative actions, employment issues, and discrimination issues. Sites with a chat room in which you can ask peers about their experience might be especially valuable if you live in a rural area. Once you connect with the information available, links will take you to many other sites, some of which may pertain to your particular experience. Check them out.

Suggested Websites to Begin Your Search

Self Help for Hard of Hearing People
www.hearingloss.org (or)
www.SHHH.org

Alexander Graham Bell Association for the
Deaf and Hard of Hearing
http://www.agbell.org/

Association of Late Deafened Adults
www.ALDA.org

Better Hearing Institute
www.bhi.org

Hear-It
http://www.hear-it.org/

House Ear Institute
www.hei.org

League for the Hard of Hearing
www.lhh.org

Other Hearing Related Websites

Hearing Education and Awareness for Rockers
www.hearnet.com

Cochlear Implant Association Inc
http://www.cici.org/

Audiology Information Websites

American Speech-Language-Hearing Association
www.ASHA.org

American Academy of Audiology
www.audiology.com

Virtual Tour of the Ear
http://ctl.augie.edu/perry/perry.htm

Employment Support Websites

Vocational Rehabilitation Offices by State
http://www.jan.wvu.edu/SBSES/VOCREHAB.HTM

Job Accommodation Network
http://janweb.icdi.wvu.edu/
800-526-7234

Captioned Movies Websites

National Center for Accessible Media
http://ncam.wgbh.org/mopix/nowshowing.html

Insight Cinema
http://insightcinema.org/

COPING SKILLS TRAINING

Coping skills training is a must for you and close family members. Unfortunately classes are rare and much of your training may need to come from books. However, taking a class where you have an opportunity to discuss issues with others is important. If one does not already exist in your community, ask your local audiologists, medical clinics, mental health clinics, or school speech therapists if they can provide the community such a class. If not, read a few of the basic hearing loss books and instruct a class yourself. By teaching a class you will soon become the expert. Keep in mind, those you are instructing know less than you do. Invite in an audiogolist or hearing aid dispenser to discuss hearing loss and hearing aids; these professionals will often appreciate the free publicity opportunity. The purpose of the class is to educate people on the basics, make them aware of resources, and provide a place to share their experience. Often classes result in an on-going support group.

SUPPORT GROUPS

If you have a local support group, I highly encourage you to attend at least three to five meetings. Meet other people who share your experience. They may be the only ones who intimately understand your frustrations and challenges. Sharing out loud what you are feeling and thinking will release blocked energy and help you to deal positively with your hearing loss. Support group partici- pants can refer you to doctors and suggest good hearing aids and other assistive listening devices. Members can support you through everyday hearing-loss challenges including surgery and asking for accommodations at your church, doctor's office, place of employment, or at- torney's office. Asking for accommodations is stressful. I highly recommend that you find two to five people who share your experience with whom you can talk about your challenges and from whom you can seek support.

I started a support group at my church and even though the members don't meet regularly, they know they have a voice with the church to represent their ac- commodation needs on the platform and in classes. They also feel connected with one another and know they have other people with whom they can share as personal needs arise.

Suggested National Organizations

Self Help for Hard of Hearing People
www.SHHH.org (or)
www.hearingloss.org
7910 Woodmont Ave., Suite 1200
Bethesda, MD 20814
301-657-2248

Association of Late Deafened Adults
www.ALDA.org

LIP READING CLASSES

I strongly recommend that you take a lip reading or a speech reading class to develop your "third ear." (Lip reading focuses exclusively on reading lips, whereas speech reading classes teach you to read other body language clues as well.) After even a concentrated three weeks of training you will develop your "third ear" and begin to relax when conversing with others. Learning how to lip/speech read just a little can make your life much less stressful. Students report that their greatest joy is not asking others to repeat themselves. It will also help family and friends when they feel you relax and not struggling to participate in conversations. Fortunately the sounds most people can't hear, are easy to lip read.

You can hire a speech therapist to instruct you individually but the cost is prohibitive for most people. Find a class, or make one happen in your community. Check your local community adult education schools and any centers for Deaf training to find a lip reading class. If you can't locate a class, check with speech therapists at your school system. Ask them to arrange a training class in your area. My church was willing to sponsor a lip reading class when I located a speech therapist to volunteer to instruct it. (Since the class, she advocated within her school's adult education program and they now offer a lip reading class to the general public.)

CLOSED CAPTIONING:
TELEVISION AND MOVIES

All televisions manufactured since 1993 have a built-in closed captioning unit. Activate the technology in your television to try it out. It isn't perfect and it takes a while to get used to it, but for many people it's better than not having it.

In many metropolitan centers, movie theatres have limited showings of movies that are closed captioned. Generally the showings are during the day. Contact your local theatre(s). If they do not show any closed captioned movies, ask them if they could for limited showings and invite any senior groups and/or Deaf groups. A regular group of viewers might even help the theatre make the selections.

ACCOMMODATIONS IN PUBLIC PLACES

Every theater, hotel, and public meeting room, including courtrooms, are required by law to provide some sort of listening devices when requested. Frequently it will be an FM system that channels sound from the P.A. system through an FM receiver and an ear bud placed in your ear.

If you require such equipment when you travel, call the facility ahead to request access to the equipment. Experience shows that not all facilities have them; if they are missing in your community, advocate for them. If your hearing is such that you require a live captioner, especially in courtrooms, call ahead to make arrangements.

One woman discovered that a local hospital did not offer closed captioning on its televisions. She advocated for it, hospital technicians made the minor adjustments and now all patients can get closed captioning when requested.

Advocating in your community for accommodations can become an on-going pursuit. Another woman discovered at her hospital that a breast cancer prevention video was provided for patients. When she asked for it with captioning, it was not available. She advocated for it, insisting that the audience most at risk were senior women, and the hospital made available a closed captioned version. I've heard many stories about one person requesting a change and the power of that one person to make an accommodation available for all who need it.

HEARING EAR DOGS

Just as seeing-eye dogs assist people who are blind, hearing-ear dogs are trained to assist people who are Deaf or hard of hearing. They are trained to alert you to door knocks, someone coming into your office, and various indications of danger, and they provide wonderful companionship. You can find out more information by contacting the following organizations:

International Hearing Dog, Inc.
5901 East 89th
Henderson, CO 80640
303-287-3277

Dogs for the Deaf
10175 Wheeler Rd
Central Point, OR 97502
503-826-9220

Hearing Ear Dogs of Canada
1154 Highway W
Ancaster, ONT L9G 3K9
416-648-1522
416-648-2262(TDD)

As is true of everything in life, the more we give, the more we receive. Check out these resources to transform your experience of hearing loss.

Improving Communication

With one out of every ten people experiencing a loss in their hearing, it takes a community to support a hearing loss. The best thing we can do to encourage family and friends to support us with our hearing loss is to educate them. Most people don't know what to do. This section offers a variety of thoughtful suggestions that could greatly improve and empower our interpersonal communication. Before taking action, read this section first and become familiar with the tips and their benefits; as you decide which help with your hearing loss. Invite friends or family members to read over this chapter, then discuss which tips are important. Ask your supporter how hearing loss has impacted communication between you. Share with them your own observations (ie. you don't hear "sh" sounds, you don't hear high sounds like a child's voice, you don't hear any words if there's music on in the background). This will begin a dialogue and encourage them to share as much as they know and understand about hearing loss.

For some, it may be difficult to openly share with others who might not understand what it's like to miss half a conversation. On the other hand, offering this information to someone can be a heartfelt way to reach out. In either case, we need to be receptive, caring, generous, and patient with ourselves as we teach loved ones about our loss and train them to be part of the growing community of "hearing loss" supporters.

APPROACHING SOMEONE WITH HEARING LOSS

When you encounter people with hearing loss, you can best support them by asking how you can be more sensitive to their loss and the specific challenges they face. If they are comfortable with their loss and not self-conscious about asking for assistance, they will suggest ways to help. If their hearing loss is new to them, they may be too shy to ask, or they may not yet fully understand how it impacts them, making it difficult to connect. In situations like this, you can learn from them by observing, experimenting and asking questions that will reveal their specific problem allowing you to then recognize the degree of hearing loss.

Since everyone's hearing loss is different, you need to be aware of some of the basic signs. Some people can't hear high sounds, such as a child's voice, whereas some can't hear the low sound of a man's voice. Some can't distinguish between the sounds of "f" and "s". Some have a mild hearing loss while others may have a severe hearing loss.

The first indication of hearing loss in others usually appears when a reply or comment doesn't correspond to what was originally said. In fact, you may have already experienced a few "nonsense answers" from the person sharing this information with you. For example, I may say, "Let's go to the mall," and my friend, thinking I said, "Let's call Paul," may answer, "Paul's not home, he's at his uncle's house." To me, this answer makes no sense. "Nonsense answers" indicate a hearing loss.

Many people with hearing loss only hear parts of words. I may say, "I'm going to the lake next summer." They may hear, "I oh to a ake text umer." By missing certain sounds and/or mishearing words, they do not receive the whole message. To fill in the missing pieces, their brain works overtime, interfering with their ability to communicate and adding to their frustration.

The following tips give additional ways friends and family can assist those with hearing loss to fill in the missing pieces of the puzzle and communicate with confidence. By using these simple tips, you can make a huge difference in their life.

TIPS TO IMPROVE YOUR COMMUNICATION

1. Speak into their best ear.

Most people with hearing loss have one ear that hears better than the other. Ask which one that is and be sure always to speak into that ear.

2. Get the person's attention before you speak.

People with hearing loss need to know that you're speaking to them. The worst thing you can do is to talk to them from another room. The best thing you can do is to face them and maintain eye contact while talking. This way they will know you are talking.

3. Keep your mouth visible and empty when speaking.

People with hearing loss learn quickly to read lips so they can pick up clues to the sounds they miss. Remove any obstacle from in front of your mouth or in your mouth. When they see your mouth, they can read your lips and tell the difference between words like "L"ake, "B"ake or "F"ake. (Look in a mirror to see how you can see these clues on your own lips.)

4. Speak clearly at a moderate pace.

People with hearing loss need "white space" or silence between each sound they hear in order to give their brain time to fill in the missing sounds. When you speak clearly, they can hear the sound better. When you speak at a moderate pace, they have time to detect clues that fill in the missing sounds.

Try this experiment. Read this sentence out loud and as fast as you can: "I'm going to the beach next summer and my cousin Ray is going to teach me to surf!" Saying all those words fast makes it hard for a hearing person to understand. Can you hear how difficult it is? Repeat the sentence at your regular pace, saying each word clearly. Can you hear the "white space" in between each sound? This white space gives them extra time for their brain to fill in the missing sounds.

5. Speak at a normal volume.

If your voice has a normal volume, use it. However, if you happen to have a soft voice, it helps for you to speak up or "project" your voice. To project your voice, you will need to assert more energy behind it as when actors project their voice from the stage so the audience can hear them. Projecting, however, is not shouting. Shouting is actually not good for people with hearing loss and can make it more difficult for them to comprehend what you're saying. Here's how it works. When you say a word, you send out a sound wave. This is what the ears use to signal the brain that a word has been said. Shouting distorts or changes the sound wave. It's almost the same as saying a different word. People are accustomed to hearing words spoken a certain way. Practice it yourself. Say "Look at my book" at a normal volume, then shout it. Was it easier or harder to understand when you shouted?

6. Use facial expressions and common gestures.

We read the body language of others to get the whole message. If a friend says to you, without using facial expressions and gestures, "I'm going to the mountains," you might not know if he was excited about going. But if his face is bright and his hand points to the mountains, you know he is excited. People with hearing loss depend on nonverbal clues to fill in sounds they cannot hear.

7. Let people know when you change the subject.

Conversations among friends or family are often lively and can easily lead from one topic to another without any warning or for no reason at all. People with hearing loss, however, aren't able to "shift gears" as readily and may not be aware that the subject has changed. Then quickly they realize the clues they hear/see no longer support the subject they thought was being discussed, and soon feel left out and left behind. It will take a special effort on your part to be sure they understand the new subject you are discussing.

One way to notify people with hearing loss that the topic has changed is to get their attention and give a quick summary statement and/or question. For example, when you and your friends start talking about camping last summer and you notice that your friend with hearing loss seems to have lost track of the conversation, give her a clue about the change in subject by asking someone else in the group a question that requires a specific answer, such as: "Ben, how many days were you and your church group at Lake Shasta last summer?"

This lets the person with hearing loss know that the discussion is about Ben's trip last summer. It's often confusing for people with hearing loss to follow topic changes. You can be of great help to them by making sure they stay "connected" with the conversation.

8. Rephrase or use different words if necessary.

When a person with a hearing loss can't hear the specific sounds in a word (like "m" or "n" sounds), it often does no good to repeat the word. It's better to use a different word or a different sentence with different sounds. These additional sounds will give your friend more clues to help her understand your message. For instance, if "Let's go to the mall" wasn't heard correctly, what else could you say to get the message across? You could say, "Would you like to go to Wal-Mart?" Or, "I want to go shopping, let's go to the Town & Country Mall." You'll have a better chance of being understood by giving a variety of clues as opposed to just repeating the same word or sound she may not be able to hear.

ADVANCED TIPS
TO IMPROVE YOUR COMMUNICATION

Once you become comfortable using the above tips, here are some additional tips that will help you and your family or friends communicate with a person who has hearing loss.

1. Talk in a well-lit and quiet environment.
At large gatherings, find a quiet place to sit and talk alone. The less background noise, the easier it is to hear. Also, select a place that has good lighting so your face can be seen clearly. If there's a sunny window or bright light, have the person with hearing loss sit with the light source behind his back. If you sit in front of the light, your face will be in the shadow and he won't be able to see your face because he'll be "blinded" by the glare of the light behind you. Remember, in order to read your lips, people with hearing loss need to see your mouth as well as identify your facial expressions.

2. Plan ahead for special situations.
Certain places present a variety of obstacles to communication. When dining in a restaurant, for example, in my experience it works best for people with hearing loss to wait until everyone else has ordered and all the specific questions have been answered. This allows the server to give the person with hearing loss his full attention. Then the person with hearing loss can state her order in

full, giving all the pertinent details, as in: "I'll have the 3-egg special, eggs sunnyside up, with sausages and dry whole-wheat toast and a small orange juice." This kind of planning avoids the situations in which the server needs to keep asking questions that the person with hearing loss won't be able to hear easily.

If people with hearing loss are going to a movie, a hotel or other public place, suggest they ask to use the "FM" system. An FM system is an Assistive Listening Device (ALD) that, like a small, personal FM radio station, connects the speaker to the listener, who can adjust the volume as needed. Public places are required by law to provide an amplification system when asked to do so. This device amplifies the sound at a movie, or the volume of a speaker or lecturer, and looks like a small radio with earphones or like your personal CD player. Most places will have this specific device but it may be necessary to call ahead to make special arrangements. For more details on other types of ALD's, a number of websites provide extensive information.

3. Encourage people with hearing loss to express their hearing needs.

Strangers won't automatically know what to do to help those with hearing loss to understand them. They will usually oblige and offer to help, but without training or knowledge of what to do, they often feel helpless. Encourage your friends or family members with hearing loss to tell others what they can do to help them to communicate better. Most people with hearing loss learn to say, "I have a hearing loss. Please face me and speak clearly so I can understand you. Thank you."

Occasionally if others are being rude or it's really noisy, I will speak up to clarify what the person with hearing loss needs. It's always best, however, if this person is the one who does the asking.

4. Write down key words.

Some words are hard to understand, like Honolulu (where its sounds come from the back of the throat-say it and see!) or medical terms that are unfamiliar. Numbers (as in phone numbers and addresses) are easy to misunderstand, too. Encourage people with hearing loss always to carry a pad and pencil and to ask that phone numbers, addresses, calendar dates and spelling of uncommon names be written down.

Remember, communicating with someone with hearing loss takes a special effort. You need to remember to face them, speak clearly, and say things using different words if necessary. But as friend or family, it's worth staying connected with them. Your love will show when you use these tips.

ABOUT THE AUTHOR

Susan Roberts, raised by a mother with a severe to profound hearing loss, currently volunteers for the Agency for Hearing in Sacramento, California, where she facilitates their "Living with Hearing Loss" coping skills class and advocates for people with hearing loss. She is also active in Unity, a New Thought organization. Her website is: www.susanlroberts.com.

Thank You!

. . . for selecting this book from
DeVorss Publications.
If you would like to receive a complete catalog
of our specialized selection of current and
classic Metaphysical, Spiritual, Inspirational,
Self-Help, and New Thought books,
please visit our website or
give us a call and ask for your free copy.

DeVorss Publications
www.devorss.com
800-843-5743